Real Food For Pregnancy

AN EMPOWERING COMPANION
ON THE ROAD TO
MOTHERHOOD

Helen Clayton

Table of content

Introduction

In the realm of health and well-being, a culinary awakening is underway, and at its heart lies the concept of "Real Pregnancy Food." In a world where nurturing the journey of motherhood is both an art and a science, the spotlight is turning towards a gastronomic revolution designed to nourish and delight expectant mothers.

Real pregnancy food goes beyond mere sustenance; it is a celebration of life's most precious moments, crafted with care to provide essential nutrients and wholesome flavors. This culinary approach acknowledges the unique nutritional needs of pregnant women, blending science with the art of gastronomy to create a symphony of tastes that resonate with both health and indulgence.

In this culinary landscape, vibrant fruits, leafy greens, and whole grains converge to create dishes that are not only delicious but also rich in the vital elements that support a healthy pregnancy. From nutrient-packed salads to hearty and comforting meals, real pregnancy food is a testament to the belief that nourishment during this transformative period can be both enjoyable and beneficial. Join us on a journey where each bite is a step towards nurturing life, where the culinary canvas is painted with the hues of health, and where real pregnancy food becomes a flavorful ode to the incredible miracle of motherhood.

Concept of real pregnancy food

A wholesome, well-balanced meal designed especially to suit the nutritional demands of expectant mothers is referred to as "real pregnancy food." A woman's body changes significantly during pregnancy, and the growing baby needs certain nutrients for healthy growth and development. The goal of real pregnancy food is to supply these essential nutrients for the mother's health as well as the baby's healthy development.

Key components of a real pregnancy diet include:

Folate and Folic Acid: These B-vitamins are essential for protecting the growing fetus against neural tube abnormalities. Citrus fruits, legumes, fortified cereals, and leafy green vegetables are foods high in folate.

Calcium: Found in dairy products, leafy greens, and fortified plant-based milk substitutes, calcium is necessary for the growth of the baby's bones and teeth.

Iron: To sustain their growing blood volume and avoid anemia, pregnant women frequently require higher levels of iron. Lean meats, chicken, fish, beans, and iron-fortified cereals are good sources of iron.

Protein: Essential for the development of the baby's tissues, protein comes from dairy products, eggs, fish, poultry, lean meats, legumes, and nuts.

Omega-3 Fatty Acids: Found in walnuts, flaxseeds, chia seeds, and fatty fish (such as salmon and trout), omega-3 fatty acids are essential for the development of the baby's brain and eyes.

Vitamins and Minerals: A range of fruits and vegetables include vital vitamins (like C) and minerals (such potassium and magnesium) required for general development and well-being.

Hydration: It's important to maintain adequate hydration during pregnancy. Although water is the ideal beverage, other options for staying hydrated include herbal teas and some fruits that are high in water.
Pregnant women should speak with medical

specialists so that their food regimens can be customized for their unique needs and any potential difficulties. Furthermore, it is frequently advised to abstain from specific foods and substances (such as raw fish, unpasteurized dairy, and high caffeine) in order to protect the mother and the unborn baby. Real pregnancy food promotes a healthy, balanced diet that benefits the unborn baby's development as well as the expectant mother's.

Chapter One

Understanding nutritional needs

One of the best things you can do when pregnant is to eat healthily. As your pregnancy goes on, eating a healthy diet will help you meet your body's increasing needs. The objective is to strike a balance between keeping a healthy weight and obtaining adequate nutrients to promote the growth of your baby.

Your baby's growth and development will be aided by a nutritious diet during pregnancy. Recognize which nutrients are most important to you and where to get them.

The fundamentals of a healthy diet hold true throughout pregnancy: consume an abundance of fruits, vegetables, whole grains, lean protein, and healthy fats. Nonetheless, certain nutrients in a pregnant woman's diet need particular consideration. And this is what comes in first.

Folate and folic acid.

Prevent birth defects of the brain and spinal cord using folate and folic acid.
One B vitamin that helps avoid major issues with the growing brain and spinal cord is folate (also known as neural tube abnormalities). Folic acid is the name for the synthetic version of folate that can be found in fortified foods and supplements. It has been demonstrated that taking folic acid supplements reduces the chance of preterm birth and low birth weight babies.

How much you need: 400 micrograms (mcg) of folic acid or folate per day prior to conception, and 600–1,000 mg per day during pregnancy

Sources: Fortified cereals are excellent providers of folic acid. Natural sources of folate include citrus fruits, dark green leafy vegetables, and dry beans, peas, and lentils.

Calcium: Builds stronger bones.

For healthy bones and teeth, both you and your baby need calcium. Additionally, calcium promotes the neurological, muscular, and circulatory systems' optimal operation.

How much you need: 1000mg/day while Teenagers who are pregnant require 1,300mg/day

Sources: The best absorbed sources of calcium are dairy products. Among the non dairy sources are kale and broccoli. A lot of fruit juices and cereals for breakfast also contain calcium fortification.

Vitamin D: Encourage strong bones

Together with calcium, vitamin D aids in the development of your baby's teeth and bones.

How much you need: each day is 600 international units (IU).

Sources: Salmon and other fatty fish are excellent sources of vitamin D. Orange juice and fortified milk are further alternatives.

Protein: Encourage development

Protein is essential to the growth of your

unborn baby throughout pregnancy.

How much you need: 71 grams (g) daily.

Sources: Excellent sources of protein include eggs, shellfish, poultry, and lean meat. Nuts, seeds, beans and peas, and soy products are further options.

Iron: Prevent anemia caused by a lack of iron.

Hemoglobin is made by the body using iron. The red blood cells' hemoglobin protein transports oxygen to the body's tissues. You require twice as much iron during pregnancy as non-pregnant women do. In order to produce enough blood to give your unborn baby oxygen, your body requires this iron. Iron deficiency anemia may arise if there is insufficient iron in your body stores or if you receive insufficient iron during pregnancy. You may get fatigue or headaches. In addition to raising the risk of postpartum depression, low birth weight babies, and early birth, severe iron deficiency anemia during pregnancy also raises these risks.

How much you need: 27 milligrams each day.

Sources: Fish, chicken, and lean red meat are excellent providers of iron. Other alternatives are veggies, legumes, and morning cereals enriched with iron.

Food aversions and cravings

You may develop food aversions during pregnancy, which means you won't enjoy the flavor or aroma of certain foods. Additionally, you might be desiring one or more food kinds.

Pregnancy Cravings

You may find yourself yearning for a donut, Chinese food, or an unusual mashup such as the traditional pickles and ice cream.

The reason behind food aversions or desires in pregnant women is unknown. Nonetheless, scientists think hormones are involved.

It's acceptable to occasionally give in to these cravings, particularly if they are for items that are included in a balanced diet. Nonetheless, you ought to make an effort to consume fewer processed and junk food items.

Usually, there's a delicious substitute that's a better choice. Do you have a craving for fries? With so many beneficial elements, oven-roasted sweet potato wedges can feel just as decadent.

Pregnancy aversions

Conversely, food aversions might only become an issue if they pertain to meals that are critical to a baby's growth and development.
If you have negative side effects from foods you should be eating during pregnancy, consult your doctor. To make up for the nutrients you're not getting enough of in your diet, your doctor may recommend additional meals or supplements.

Pica

A disease called pica results in desires for foods that are nutritionally worthless. Among other weird foods, pregnant women with pica may wish to consume clay, cigarette ashes, or starch.

A pregnant lady experiencing pica may be experiencing a vitamin or mineral deficiency. If you have cravings for or have consumed nonfood products, it's critical to let your doctor know. Consuming such foods might be harmful to both you and your
baby.

Chapter Two

Tailoring diets to pregnancy stages

A balanced diet is crucial for fulfilling the physical demands of pregnancy and enhancing fetal health. Whole grains, fruits, vegetables, and iron-rich diets can all be good, but alcohol, caffeine, and some fish and cheeses may not be safe.

Expectant mother's diet should have a balance of proteins, carbs, and fats to ensure a successful pregnancy.

First trimester

Welcome to the first trimester of pregnancy! This is an exciting and maybe a bit scary time. And sometimes, the excitement of seeing a positive test is quickly thwarted by the entrance of morning sickness, exhaustion, breast pain and heartburn.

Before you even see a positive test, your body

is already changing. And even though pregnancy is a special time for most expecting mothers, the physical symptoms can be a real drag.

What is actually going on in your body during those first 13 weeks, which foods to eat in the first trimester to get the nutrients you and your baby need, and what to do if you feel sick from sunup to sundown.

Folic acid is an important vitamin that helps prevent neural tube defects. Women need to take at least 400 micrograms of folic acid daily starting at least one month prior to conception and throughout the duration of the pregnancy. Folic acid is found in dietary supplements like your daily prenatal pill and is added to fortified grains, including breakfast cereal, bread, pasta and rice.

Folate is the naturally occurring form of the vitamin found mainly in dark green vegetables such as broccoli, asparagus and romaine lettuce and in other plant foods, including avocado, beans and oranges.

The baby eats what you eat and needs vitamins and minerals to support the growth of its brain and body, however tiny. Karges notes that key nutrients during the first trimester to support a healthy pregnancy include calcium (1,000 milligrams/day), folate (600 mcg/day) and iron (27 mg/day). "These increased nutrient needs can typically be met by eating a diet that offers a wide variety of healthy foods and supplementing with a prenatal vitamin."

"Because your baby's nervous system is starting to develop, it is also important to get adequate amounts of choline, B12 and omega-3 fatty acids," adds Ingrid Anderson, RDN, founder of Simply Confident Nutrition. "Sources of these nutrients include eggs, salmon and walnuts."

Although your body is hard at work, you do not need any extra calories until the second trimester unless you're carrying multiples (twins, triplets or more). According to the

women carrying one baby may gain between 1 and 5 pounds during the first trimester.

First-trimester weight gain may be due to increased blood and fluid volume, as long as you're not overeating.

Second trimester

Congratulations! You made it to the second trimester of pregnancy. You can take a deep breath and relax. The risk of miscarriage has dropped dramatically, and you are hopefully coming out of the fog of exhaustion and morning sickness.

.. While some pregnant women may experience health issues throughout their pregnancy, the worst should have passed. The second trimester is the best, according to veteran moms, because the extreme fatigue and sickness have faded but you are yet to feel the (physical) weight of the baby.

You have fantastic news! You can now eat a larger meal. To promote your baby's growth and development throughout the second trimester, you should consume an additional 340 calories every day.

However, avoid "eating for two" otherwise you may gain unhealthy amounts of weight, which could have negative effects on both you and your unborn baby. Not to add that after delivery, you will have to lose more the more you gain.

There is no need to count calories, though. Focus on food groups, not numbers. According to dietitian Molly Cleary, R.D. of New York-Presbyterian Hospital, "foods that are high in calories but won't have detrimental effects on your blood sugar and cholesterol include avocados, nuts (like walnuts or almonds) and nut butters, seeds (like pumpkin seeds or ground flaxseeds), unsweetened dried fruits, and hummus." Iron is also important, she says. "Try getting your iron from at least one serving of seafood or poultry, a half cup of beans, and at least one serving of leafy greens daily. Bonus points for consuming vitamin C-rich foods like citrus fruits and red bell peppers along with your plant-based iron." Iron is better absorbed when vitamin C is present. "Calcium is also of particular concern," according to her, "It can be found in dairy (such as yogurt and low-fat milk), other fortified milk substitutes and leafy greens."

According to Karges, the development of the baby's skeleton and brain during the second trimester also depends on vitamin D, magnesium, and omega-3 fats. For the duration of your pregnancy, keep taking your prenatal vitamins.

Third Trimester

You're nearing the end of the third trimester. It is anticipated that the baby will arrive in about 12 weeks. It's possible that you're not feeling the well-known Braxton-Hicks contractions. Don't panic if you aren't having every symptom that has been reported online. Every woman is different. Go on dates and take things easy, but don't forget to eat healthily. The infant is still developing. What's going on and how to properly fuel your body are explained here.

The baby is mostly developed by now, but don't let that be a reason to cut back on your workout and nutritious diet. A vital period for the development of the lungs and bones is the third trimester.

Additionally, and fortunately, the baby is gaining weight! "During the third trimester, babies gain the majority of their weight while mom's breasts enlarge in preparation for nursing and her blood volume continues to rise.
Make sure you're receiving enough iron from food and supplements (only as directed by a doctor), as babies store up the majority of the

iron they'll need for the first few months after birth during the last trimester, advises Tolbert. "You'll find iron in foods like leafy greens, beans, meat and poultry. To improve absorption, try to eat foods strong in vitamin C together with foods high in iron whenever possible, the expert advice. Vitamin C is abundant in red bell peppers, kale, oranges, and strawberries.

Include omega-3s in your shopping list as well. Good fats can be found in foods including flaxseed, walnuts, salmon, tuna, and chia seeds. Two omega-3 fatty acids found in fish, DHA and EPA, help a baby's brain develop normally. Furthermore, a 2016 study that was published in the New England Journal of Medicine discovered that EPA and DHA consumption during pregnancy may lower the likelihood that your unborn child may have asthma. A daily fish oil supplement taken by expectant mothers during the third trimester reduced the child's risk of developing asthma by thirty percent between the ages of three and five. However, before using any supplements, speak with your doctor. Additionally, keep taking your prenatal vitamins for the duration of your pregnancy.

If your pregnancy has lasted longer than 40 weeks, you probably want to know how to induce labor. "Every family and culture has its own traditions and folklore around labor-inducing foods-but there's no hard proof any of them work," Tolbert asserts. As an alternative, she advises "considering adding dates to your diet in your last trimester." "There's some research suggesting they help ripen your cervix, which might speed up labor once it starts. Studies show that consuming dates in the last two to four weeks before delivery promotes cervical softening. However, in one trial, this benefit was only observed in women who consumed six dates per day. Consult your doctor before moving on, especially if you have gestational diabetes, as one date contains eighteen grams of carbohydrates.

Chapter Three

Crafting real pregnancy food

A nutritious, well-balanced diet is essential for the health of expectant mothers and their unborn babies. While there isn't a one-size-fits-all approach to pregnant nutrition, there are a few important ideas to remember when eating.

What is Real Food

Eating "real food" is often regarded as a healthful habit. The concept of "real food," however, is a murky one in the field of nutrition. Here are several methods for assessing how "real" your diet is.

Foods high in nutrients, also called nutrient-dense foods, are nutrient-rich. There are two categories for nutrients: macronutrients, such as proteins, lipids, and carbs; and micronutrients, such as vitamins and minerals.

A food is deemed nutrient-rich if it contains high levels of vitamins, minerals, fiber, protein, and/or beneficial fatty acids. Conversely, food is regarded as nutrient-poor if it lacks many of these ingredients. The majority of real foods are high in nutrients and support bodily nourishment.

Whole foods are foods eaten in a manner consistent with their natural state. The majority of whole foods are free of artificial additives, processed carbs, added sugars, added tastes, or colors. Real foods include fruits, vegetables, dairy, meat, poultry, and fish, as well as nuts, seeds, beans, and other naturally high-nutrient foods. Majority of whole foods are naturally nutrient-dense

Unprocessed foods areLike whole foods, they do not undergo any modifications and have a natural appearance. Many foods in modern society are processed to the point where they are hardly distinguishable from their natural state and do not meet the definition of a real food.

Why Eat Real Food While Pregnant?

Eating full, nutrient-dense foods provides your

body with the nutrition it needs to develop into a healthy baby. Your baby's health will be at its best as a result of your healthy diet and nutrient reserves as a parent. In addition to lowering the risk of pregnancy issues like gestational diabetes, hypertension (high blood pressure), and premature labor, real foods also aid in preventing anemia throughout pregnancy. Making dietary adjustments throughout pregnancy aids in the healing process after giving birth.

A Well Balanced Pregnancy Diet

These ideas might help you create a balanced, healthful pregnancy diet. A healthy diet should include meals and snacks that are well-balanced for everyone, but it becomes even more crucial during pregnancy. In general, a good method to nourish your body throughout pregnancy is to incorporate actual foods into filling meals and snacks.

Eat a diversified diet rich in nutrient-dense foods, such as:

 fruits and vegetables for fiber and vitamins. Complex carbs for fiber, iron, B vitamins, and folate.

Lean proteins to promote the best possible growth and development for your infant.
Good fats help your baby's brain development and satisfy your energy needs.

During pregnancy, several micronutrients become significantly more crucial.

Vitamin A is important for your baby's vision and immune system, among other minerals.
Vitamin D for the growth of your baby's bones.
To develop your baby's teeth, bones, muscles, heart, and nerves, calcium must combine with vitamin D.
Choline for the brain development of your infant.
Folate supports the growth of your baby's brain and spinal cord.
Iron to help your growing blood supply as a prospective mother.

Easy Modifications

Knowing what things to consume and what to avoid is as beneficial as knowing what to eat. In general, everyone benefits from reducing processed foods, but pregnant women who want to optimize their diets should take particular note of this. Make minor adjustments within each food group to make your diet more genuinely centered on real foods rather than attempting to exclude entire food groupings.

The foods that are highest in nutrients are entire fruits and vegetables. Frozen fruits and veggies are a fantastic alternative as they keep their nutrients intact. Dried fruit without added sugar also offers healthy nutrients. To stay away from extra sugars, make sure to search for products that are unsweetened and have no added sugar. You should restrict your intake of fruit snacks, veggie chips, and other processed meals that appear to contain fruits and vegetables but actually don't.

Whole grains and refined grains are the two main types of carbohydrates. Brown rice, quinoa, oats, and whole-wheat bread and pasta are examples of whole grains. These grains have undergone less processing and are higher in healthy components. White bread, spaghetti, and rice are examples of refined grains; they are less nutrient-dense and highly processed. Make an effort to select whole grains wherever you can.

The least processed proteins are usually thought to be the healthiest choices. Reducing the amount of processed meats (sausage, bacon) in your diet can enhance its overall quality.During pregnancy, lean beef or pig chops, chicken, and shellfish are all excellent sources of protein. Beans and other plant-based proteins like tofu are also healthful options.

Dairy products and eggs are also nutritious, complete foods that are useful during pregnancy. Eating whole-milk dairy products and eggs can also enhance nutritional intake in general. One of the few foods high in choline, which is essential for the development of your baby's brain, is eggs. The most amount of choline is obtained from eating the entire egg. Full-fat, whole-milk dairy gives your body the fat it needs to absorb A, D, E, and K vitamins.

An essential component of your total energy requirements throughout pregnancy is healthy fats. More specifically, the proper development of the fetal brain depends on omega-3 fatty acids. More precisely, docosahexaenoic acid (DHA), an omega-3 fatty acid, is essential for the development of your baby's brain. During pregnancy, avocados, nuts, seeds, and fatty seafood are excellent sources of good fats. Even though fish and shellfish are excellent providers of iron, healthy fats, and protein, pregnant women should be cautious when consuming some kinds of seafood because they may contain high levels of mercury.

Being Realistic

While following these suggestions would be ideal, receiving the nutrition your body requires during pregnancy may be more difficult. Cravings for certain foods are normal and might affect your eating choices all during pregnancy. Food aversions are also prevalent, and at certain stages of your pregnancy, you might not be able to eat some of the foods you know are healthful.

Your prenatal vitamin is an essential component in making sure you are getting the nutrients you need, even if it isn't a meal and doesn't matter what you eat on a daily basis. Prenatal vitamins make sure you and your unborn baby get the nutrition you need on a daily basis during pregnancy. Nonetheless, the elements found in food work in concert with one another, thus obtaining your nutrients from food is usually preferable than taking supplements. Take your prenatal as usual, but try your best to consume a range of real meals as well. See your physician or nutritionist if you require assistance selecting a prenatal vitamin.

Chapter Four

Incorporating superfoods

Nothing motivates you to eat healthier than learning what you are expecting. Following all, your body is undergoing significant changes, and to be healthy and strong, you and your unborn baby require an abundance of vitamins and nutrients. But what exactly qualifies as a pregnancy-safe diet? Rest assured, we've got you covered. Here are ten pregnancy-friendly meals along with their corresponding benefits.

Eggs

What it has: Eggs are the best source of protein during pregnancy, regardless of how you choose to prepare them—fried, scrambled, hard-boiled, or omelet-style. They are also an excellent source of iron, choline, and folate.

Why it benefits you both equally: Eggs are a convenient, adaptable, and reasonably priced source of protein. They also include choline. Never heard about the last one? In addition to lowering the incidence of neural tube abnormalities like spina bifida, choline is essential for the development of the fetal brain. However, because choline is found in the yolk, you must consume the entire thing to benefit from it (forget the egg-whites-only regimen).

Sweet Potatoes

What it has: Sweet potatoes are a great source of fiber, vitamin B6, potassium (even more than bananas!), iron, vitamin C, copper, and beta-carotene. Don't save them for Thanksgiving alone.

Why it benefits you both equally: While many of the nutrients found in other foods on our list are also present in sweet potatoes, we are highlighting them because they include beta-carotene, an antioxidant that your body uses to produce vitamin A. Furthermore, as you may remember, vitamin A is crucial for the growth of a baby's skin, bones, and eyes. These orange potatoes contain copper, a mineral that aids in the body's absorption of iron, and are an excellent method to meet your iron requirements. Therefore, replace your typical sides with sweet potatoes; they taste fantastic when mashed, roasted, or

French-fried.

Nuts

What they have: Packed with protein, fiber, healthy fats (including the brain-boosting omega-3s we discussed earlier), and a range of vitamins and minerals, this crunchy (and portable) snack is a powerhouse. Furthermore, eating nuts can help you receive some of the 350 mg of magnesium you should be getting now that you are pregnant.

Why you should both benefit from them: Eating meals high in magnesium promotes healthy nervous system development in the developing fetus and lowers the chance of premature labor. Keep some almond slices in your purse for a quick and easy prenatal power snack. One cup of sliced almonds has around 250 mg of magnesium. Control of cravings: Try snacking on pistachios with shells if you're feeling like a bottomless pit right now. Although they take longer to consume, they contain somewhat less magnesium (150 mg per cup), which gives your body more time to recognize when it is full.

Lentils and Beans

What they have: Beans and lentils are excellent sources of protein, iron, folate, fiber, and calcium if you're not a huge or even a meat eater. Additionally, beans—especially cooked ones—are a great source of zinc.

Why you should both benefit from them: For aspiring vegetarian and vegan mothers, beans are an excellent alternative because they contain many of the elements that are beneficial for both mom and baby when found in animal products. Additionally, beans are a great source of zinc, a necessary element that has been associated with a decreased risk of preterm birth, low birth weight, and longer labor. Do beans make you queasy? Meat, poultry, milk, fortified cereals, cashews, peas, crab, and oysters (but don't eat them raw!) are additional excellent sources of zinc.

Lean Meat

What it has: Lean beef and pork are high in iron and B vitamins in addition to being a fantastic source of protein.

Why it benefits you both equally: In order to support baby's growth and correct muscular development, your body now needs a significant increase in protein (about 25 additional grams per day). Likewise with iron: Inadequate intake of this mineral can stunt the growth of the unborn baby and raise the risk of low birth weight and premature delivery. Mom needs iron as well because it is essential for the production of red blood cells, which helps to prevent anemia. Because pregnancy causes an increase in blood volume, you should increase your iron consumption to around 27 milligrams per day. Eating meat provides a good amount of vitamins B6 and B12, which support healthy nerve and red blood cell development in the baby and reduce morning sickness in the mother.

Orange Juice

What it possesses: Have a glass of orange juice first thing in the morning to get your share of potassium, folate, and vitamin C.

Why it benefits you both equally: It's likely that you've heard a lot of talk about folic acid, or synthetic folate, which can be found in fortified foods and supplements. Try to obtain the suggested 400 micrograms of this nutrient each day as it's essential for preventing certain birth defects early in pregnancy and for maintaining a healthy pregnancy thereafter. The potassium in orange juice is essential for maintaining healthy muscles, metabolism, and general health. Due to their growing blood volume, pregnant women also require higher potassium intake, similar to iron. As you may already be aware, orange juice is a great source of vitamin C, which helps your body absorb iron more effectively, prevents colds, and maintains the health of your baby's teeth and bones. Broccoli, tomatoes, strawberries, red peppers, and other citrus fruits are good sources of vitamin C. Mangoes, another powerful food for pregnant women, have more than 20 distinct vitamins and minerals. Choose orange juice that has been fortified with vitamin D. This will help the baby's bones grow stronger by improving blood circulation in the placenta and facilitating the absorption of calcium.

Yogurt

What it has: Unexpectedly! In actuality, plain yogurt has a little bit more calcium than milk. It also contains important minerals that help form bone, like zinc, B vitamins, and protein.

Why it benefits you both equally: Eating too little calcium might be harmful to both of you because it is necessary for the development of your teeth and bones as well as for the health of your baby's. Pregnant women who want to lower their risk of low birth weight and preterm delivery should take 1,000 mg of calcium daily. Your body will take the calcium your growing child requires from your bones if your calcium level is low, which increases your chance of developing osteoporosis in the future. To get twice the protein (and fiber) in your diet, snack on Greek yogurt with fruit on top.

Oatmeal

What it has: Fiber, protein, and vitamin B6 abound in those oats.

Why it benefits you both equally: A hearty cup of oats can help you get started in the morning correctly. If you're feeling a little lethargic due to morning sickness, whole grains are fantastic for boosting your energy. Additionally, constipation is another pregnancy-related problem that all that fiber will assist with. But mom isn't the only one who profits from this. This easy breakfast recipe is also fantastic as an instant version. includes protein and vitamin B6, all of which are critical to a baby's growth. Seek for a type that has been supplemented with folic acid, iron, and B vitamins.

Leafy green

What it has: It was inevitable that these people would be on the list. Dark-green vegetables like spinach, asparagus, broccoli, and kale are packed with minerals and antioxidants, so they should be on everyone's grocery list when they're pregnant.

Why it benefits you both equally: Superfoods like these are especially crucial for expecting mothers and developing babies. This is due to the fact that leafy greens also include calcium, potassium, fiber, folate, and vitamin A in addition to all those antioxidants. Not really in the mood for spinach or asparagus? Vitamin A is also abundant in oranges.

Salmon

What it has: Omega-3 fatty acids and protein are abundant in this oily fish.

Why it benefits you both equally: To give baby a mental boost, forget about pre ordering Baby Einstein DVDs and instead make salmon a part of your diet for the next nine months. Omega-3 fatty acids, also known as DHA and EPA, are found in fish and aid in the development of the baby's brain. In fact, higher DHA levels in neonates have been linked to improved motor abilities, a lower risk of neurological disorders later in life, and a higher IQ. Not only can omega-3 fatty acids help develop a baby's vision, but salmon is also a fantastic source of lean protein for expectant mothers. Concerned about seafood? Expectant mothers are advised to limit their intake of salmon to two to three servings of four ounces or less per week due to its low mercury content. Simply not in the mood for fish right now? Eat almonds and walnuts as a snack.

Chapter Five

Healthy Pregnancy Recipes and Preparation

Indeed! These ten meals are full of nutrients and variety, perfect for a pregnancy. Please be aware that the nutritional value is an estimate that may change depending on particular components and cooking techniques. For individualized dietary guidance throughout pregnancy, always seek the advice of a healthcare provider.

1. Stuffed bell peppers with salmon and quinoa

Ingredients:
Bell peppers (a range of colors)
Cooked quinoa
Baked or grilled salmon
Spinach
Feta cheese
Olive oil
Juice from lemons
Dill (as a garnish)

Preparation:
Remove the seeds after cutting the bell
peppers in half.
In a bowl, combine the cooked quinoa, feta
cheese, sautéed spinach, and flakes salmon.
Place the mixture inside the bell peppers.
Pour in some lemon juice and olive oil.
Bake peppers until they become soft.
Place some fresh dill on top.

Nutritional Content:
25g of protein
8g of fiber
12g of fat
1.5g of omega-3 fatty acids

2. Sweet Potato and Chickpea Curry:

Ingredients

Sweet potatoes, chopped
Chickpeas, cooked
Coconuts Milk
Curry paste
Diced onion
Minced garlic
Spinach
Brown rice, if desired

Preparation:

Saute garlic and onions in a saucepan.
Curry paste, chickpeas, sweet potatoes, and
coconut milk should be added.
Once the sweet potatoes are soft, simmer
them.
Add spinach and stir until it wilts.
If preferred, serve over brown rice.

Nutritional Content:

12g of protein
10g of fiber
10g of fat
Iron: 3 milligrams

3. Black bean and Quinoa Stuffed Avocado

Ingredients:

Avocados
Cooked quinoa
Drained black beans
Corn kernels
Chopped cherry tomatoes
Lime juice

Chopped cilantro
Pepper and salt.

Preparation:

Halve the avocados and remove the pits.
In a bowl, combine quinoa, black beans, corn,
and tomatoes.
Stuff avocados full of the blend.
Sprinkle with cilantro and drizzle with lime
juice.
Add pepper and salt for seasoning.

Nutritional Content:

10g of protein
12g of fiber
15g of fat
120 micrograms of folate

4. Mango and Shrimp Salad

Ingredients

Grilled or cooked shrimp
Mixed Salad greens
Mango, sliced
Avocado, diced
Olive oil

Chopped red onion
Vinegar with balsamic
Honey
Pepper and Salt.

Preparation:

Place the salad greens on a platter.
Add red onion, avocado, mango slices, and
cooked shrimp on top.
Combine olive oil, honey, balsamic vinegar,
salt, and pepper in a whisk.
Pour the dressing over the Salad.

Nutritional Content:

18g of protein
45 mg of vitamin C
20g of good fats

5. Yogurt Parfait with Almonds and Berries

Ingredients:

Greek yogurt
Berries in combination (strawberries,
blueberries)

Sliced almonds
Honey
Granola (optional)

Preparation:

Greek yogurt can be layered in a bowl or glass.
Add the sliced almonds and mixed berries.
Pour some honey over it.
Iterate through the levels.
Add granola on top if you'd like.

Content Nutritional:

20g of protein
350 mg of calcium
6g of fiber

6. Stir-fried Turkey with Vegetables

Ingredients:

Turkey, ground
Florets of broccoli
Sliced bell peppers
Snap peas
Julienned carrots
Minced garlic
Soy sauce

Sesame oil
Brown rice, if desired

Preparation:

Ground turkey should be pan-fried until browned.
Add the bell peppers, broccoli, carrots, snap peas, and garlic.
Add sesame oil and soy sauce and stir.
Sauté the veggies until they are soft.
If preferred, serve over brown rice.

Nutritional Content:

22g of protein
7g of fiber
2.5 milligrams of iron

7. Breakfast Wrap with Egg and Spinach:

Ingredients

Whole-grain tortilla
Eggs Scrambled
Avocado, sliced
Salsa
Spinach

Feta cheese, if desired

Preparation:

Preheat the tortilla.
Top with scrambled eggs avocado slices,
salsa, feta cheese, sautéed spinach,
Roll into a wrap

Nutritional Content:

15g of protein
8g of fiber
20g of good fats

8. Vegetable and Lentil Soup

Ingredients:

Diced carrots
Rinsed Lentils
Chopped Celery
Diced Onion
Veggies broth
Minced Garlic
Diced Tomatoes
Chopped Spinach
Olive Oil
Spices and herbs (bay leaves, thyme, rose

mary)
Pepper and Salt

Preparation:

Saute garlic and onions in olive oil.
Add the veggies broth, tomatoes, celery,
carrots, and lentils.
Add spices and herbs for flavor.
Once the lentils are soft, simmer them.
Add the chopped spinach and stir.
Add pepper and salt for seasoning.

Nutritional Content:

18g of Protein
12g of fiber
4mg of Iron

9. Quinoa-topped Chicken and Vegetable Skewers

Ingredients:

Sliced chicken breast into cubes
Sliced Bell Pepper (different colors)
Cherry Tomatoes
Sliced Zucchini
Olive oil

Juice from lemons
Minced garlic
Dried Oregano's
Cooked Quinoa

Preparation:

Put the Chicken and Veggies on Skewers.
Combine the dried oregano, lemon juice,
minced garlic, and olive oil.
Apply the mixture on the skewers.
Bake or grill the chicken until cooked.
Serve on top of Cooked Quinoa.

Nutritional Content:

25g of protein
8g of fiber
10g of good fats

10. Banana and Peanut Butter Smoothie Bowl

Ingredients:

Bananas that are frozen
Peanut butter
Greek yogurt
Almond milk

Chia seeds
Granola
Strawberries cut into slices

Preparation:

Smoothly blend almond milk, peanut butter, Greek yogurt, and frozen bananas.
Transfer to a bowl.
Add sliced strawberries, granola, and chia seeds on top.

Nutritional Content:

15g of protein
10g of fiber
12g of good fats

A well-rounded and fulfilling pregnancy diet can be achieved by incorporating a range of flavors, textures, and nutrients, all of which are featured in these dishes. Adapt ingredients and quantities to suit dietary requirements and personal tastes. For individualized dietary guidance throughout pregnancy, always seek the advice of a healthcare provider.

Chapter Six

Healthy Pregnancy Meal Plan

Are you looking for a simple meal plan that is healthy and quick to prepare? Take a look at the breakfast, lunch, snack, and dinner meal plans.
You'll feel more invigorated and at ease knowing that you're providing your unborn baby with the nourishment they require for growth if you concentrate on your diet during pregnancy.

This seven-day meal plan, which incorporates snack suggestions, is based on the ideas presented in "Real Food for Pregnancy." Never forget to seek tailored guidance from a licensed dietician or healthcare professional.

Day 1:

Breakfast:

Greek yogurt parfait with almonds, mixed berries, and honey drizzled over.

Snack:

Apple slices with peanut butter

Lunch

Quinoa and black bean salad with avocado, cherry tomatoes, lime dressing.

Snack:

Hummus-topped carrot and cucumber sticks.

Dinner:

Steamed broccoli, sweet potato wedges, and baked fish marinated in lemon dill.

Day 2:

Breakfast:

Whole grain toast topped with a poached egg, mashed avocado, and chia seeds.

Snack

Greek yogurt with a small handful of granola

Lunch:

Lentil soup with a side of whole-grain roll and a mixed green salad.

Snack:

Pineapple pieces mixed with cottage cheese.

Dinner:

Brown rice topped with a stir-fried chicken and colorful veggies including bell peppers, broccoli, and snap peas.

Day 3:

Breakfast:

Whole grain bread with spinach and feta omelet .

Snack:

A handful of mixed dried fruits and nuts.

Lunch:

Whole-grain tortilla stuffed with cucumber, hummus, and leafy greens, along with turkey and vegetables.

Snack:

Cheese and whole grain crackers

Dinner:

Quinoa-stuffed bell peppers with ground turkey, black beans, tomatoes, and a side of guacamole.

Day 4:

Breakfast

Smoothie bowl that includes frozen berries, bananas, Greek yogurt, with chia seeds and granola on top.

Snack:

Almond butter on sliced pears.

Lunch

Brown rice and vegetable curry with chickpeas

Snack:

Greek yogurt topped with flaxseeds.

Dinner:

Salad of shrimp and mango dressed with a mild citrus vinaigrette, mixed greens, and avocado.

Day 5:

Breakfast:

Rolled oats, almond milk, chia seeds, banana slices, and walnuts on top of overnight oats.

Snack:

Almond and dried fruit trail mix.

Lunch:

Egg and spinach salad with cherry tomatoes, cucumber, and a balsamic vinaigrette.

Snack:

Smoothie made with Greek yogurt, spinach, banana, and a little milk.

Dinner:

Baked sweet potato with Greek yogurt on top
and a salsa of black beans and corn.

Day 6:

Breakfast

Greek yogurt with fresh berries and whole
grain pancakes

Snack:

Tzatziki and cucumber slices.

Lunch:

Tomato and basil quinoa bowl with grilled
chicken.

Snack:

Cheese slices and apple

Dinner:

Veggies and lentils stew with whole grain bread

on the side.

Day 7:

Breakfast:

Smoothie made with peanut butter, bananas, spinach, almond milk, and a dollop of protein powder

Snack:

Strawberries cut into pieces with cottage cheese.

Lunch:

Chickpeas wrap with avocado, cucumber, and tahini dressing on spinach.

Snack:

Cherry tomatoes with mozzarella balls

Dinner:

Tofu skewers and marinated veggie in a lemon-herb marinade served over quinoa.

Always remember to drink plenty of water, herbal teas, and other decaffeinated liquids to stay hydrated throughout the day. Feel free to substitute items based on dietary restrictions and personal preferences, and adjust portion proportions to suit individual needs.

What foods should I eat daily when pregnant?

The UK NHS lists a few foods that are advised to be consumed every day if you are pregnant: A minimum of five servings of fruits and vegetables, in any form—fresh, frozen, canned, dehydrated, or juiced. However, it's important to keep in mind that many fruit juices found in cartons aren't actually prepared from fresh fruit; rather, they're concentrated and may contain a high sugar content, making them less nutrient-dense.

Approximately one-third of your daily pregnancy meal plan should consist of carbohydrates, such as potatoes, rice, bread, and pasta.

Lean proteins include beef, beans, lentils, seafood (avoid mercury-filled fish), eggs (if they're prepared properly), and nuts.

Calcium-rich foods and beverages, such as dairy products, cheese, yogurt, and calcium-fortified plant milks.

Healthy Snack Options

Here are some delicious and nutrient-dense snacks to help you stick to your pregnant diet:

Edamame
Smoothie
Sliced Cheese
Nuts
Berries
Veggies with hummus or dressing
Energy balls
Banana or apple with peanut butter
Cottage cheese
Dollop sized Greek yogurt
Spread toast with almond or peanut butter.
Cereal or granola bowl with milk

What can't Expectant moms eat?

It's true that certain foods should be avoided or consumed in moderation during pregnancy since they may be unhealthy for both you and the unborn baby.

High levels of vitamin A or mercury, or the possibility of a bacterial infection, are frequently the reason for this.

Marlin
Swordfish
Uncooked fish
Uncooked meat
Processed meats, such as lunch meat and hot dogs
Liver
Uncooked eggs
Brie
Sushi
Gorgonzola
Unpasteurized cheeses
Raw milk
Energy drinks
Unwashed fruits and vegetables
Raw sprouts (such as mung beans, alfalfa, clover, or spinach)
Alcohol

Chapter Seven

Coping with common Pregnancy Discomfort

A pregnancy alters the body in numerous ways. There are changes in your body chemistry and function in addition to weight and shape. Your body secretions increase, the heart pumps harder, your body temperature rises slightly, your joints and ligaments become more flexible, and your hormones change. Changes in mood are typical and can be attributed to hormonal shifts, increased tiredness, and natural anxiety about finances, marriage duties, body image, sexuality, and becoming a parent.

The most typical pregnancy discomforts are listed below, along with some advice on how to handle them.

Nausea and vomiting

Eat little, often. During pregnancy, going too

long without food might either worsen or exacerbate nausea. Eat every one to two hours if you are constantly sick.

Steer clear of oily, high-fat foods. They are more challenging to process.

Eat dry starchy items before getting out of bed in the morning, including toast, crackers, or cereal. Additionally, it helps to remain in bed for about 20 minutes after eating and to get out of bed gradually because abruptly shifting positions might exacerbate nausea.

It may be beneficial to sip chamomile, spearmint, and peppermint teas in addition to fizzy drinks.

Consume a lot of foods high in carbohydrates, such as rice, bread, fruit, and cereal. They provide you energy and are simple to digest.

Only take prenatal vitamins as prescribed. Ask your doctor if you can skip taking them for a few weeks if they hurt your stomach.

Certain items, like tea or milk, can make a woman feel better while disturbing another. Still, most women can handle cold foods and drinks better than hot ones.

To regulate blood sugar before going to bed, eat a high-protein snack.

Don't drink too much coffee. It increases the production of acid, which may exacerbate the nausea.

Drink liquids after a 20–30 minute interval,
apart from meals.
Put on wristbands for seasickness. The
majority of pharmacies carry these.

Constipation

Eat more foods high in fiber, such as fruits, raw
vegetables, whole grain products, nuts, and
dried fruits, to increase your intake of fiber.
Pick a cereal for breakfast that provides a
minimum of 5 grams of fiber per serving. These
foods encourage regular bowel movements
and aid in softening the stool.
Have a lot of liquids.
Walking is a good kind of exercise to help ease
constipation.
Consume figs or prunes, or make prune juice.
There is a natural laxative in these fruits.
Steer clear of laxatives. Inform your healthcare
provider if the issue persists after trying the
aforementioned solutions. Prescription stool
softeners that are safe to use throughout
pregnancy are available.
Iron prescriptions might be changed if
constipation becomes an issue because iron
supplements can make it worse.

Hemorrhoids

Prevent constipation by eating a diet rich in fiber and water to help ward off hemorrhoids. The hemorrhoid region can be treated with witch hazel or Tucks pads to ease symptoms. Steer clear of OTC laxatives. Stool softeners can be taken if hard stools are making hemorrhoids worse, but first speak with your practitioner for recommendations.

Fatigue

This is a fairly typical first-trimester experience. Make the most of your rest and sleep; even quick naps will assist. After the first three months, your energy will start to increase again. However, the final few months of pregnancy are often when exhaustion and sleeplessness return. Before going to bed, unwind and prepare for sleep by having a warm bath, a massage, or a hot beverage.

Breasts tenderness

The first three months are the most noticeable for breast soreness. The breasts get bigger and sometimes very sensitive. You could feel more at ease if you wear a supportive bra.

Frequent Urination

Another pregnancy symptom that is most noticeable in the first trimester and towards the conclusion of the pregnancy is frequent urination. Don't cut back on your fluid intake in an attempt to urinate less frequently. Experiencing discomfort or burning when you urinate is normal, and the increased frequency will go away eventually.

Leg cramps

Your calf or leg cramps most often happen at night. Increasing your calcium intake could be one solution. Inquire with your doctor about calcium supplements. Stretch in bed by pointing at your heels rather than your toes. This will ease the pain of a cramp.

Heartburn

Aim for more frequent but smaller meals.
Steer clear of rich, fatty, and heavily seasoned foods.
After eating, avoid lying down completely. Use

cushions to raise your head and shoulders if you have to lie down.

Milk and carbonated drinks are common ways to relieve heartburn.

It is not advised to take some antacids when pregnant. Consult your physician before taking any over-the-counter antacid medications.

Backache

Back pain is frequently experienced during pregnancy. It results from the change in posture brought on by bearing more weight forward.

Aim to avoid being still for extended periods of time.

The most stressed lower back muscles can be strengthened and back discomfort can be reduced using an exercise known as the pelvic rock.

It will be beneficial to raise the feet while seated onto a stool.

Dizziness

Sudden changes in posture or low blood sugar might also result in dizziness or lightheadedness. To assist in preventing this emotion:

When rising from a seated or sleeping posture, take your time.
Consume healthy food often. Women who are prone to hypoglycemia should always have snacks on hand. Fruit and juices are especially healthy options.

Swelling in the hands and feets

In the final stages of pregnancy, it is typical to experience mild swelling in the hands and feet. Drinking enough water is always crucial.
Elevate your legs and feet as much as you can to help with circulation. With your knees bent, elevate your legs off the floor or bed and place them against the wall. This is a good way to empty your legs before putting on an elastic hose.

Chapter Eight

Pregnancy-related exercise

Most pregnant women should and are able to participate in mild to moderate exercise. Exercise can help you maintain your physical fitness and get your body ready for childbirth. However, before starting an exercise regimen while pregnant, talk with your healthcare provider.
During pregnancy, walking, swimming, and cycling are all great types of exercise. It is appropriate to perform strengthening workouts with light weights. Consider taking a prenatal workout class as well. Instructors are able to demonstrate safe and efficient floor activities.

Exercise's Health Benefits During Pregnancy

Pregnancy-related exercise can:
Boost endurance and strength
Bolster your muscles to get ready for labor and delivery.

Alleviate constipation
Boost physical health
Alleviate back discomfort
Boost adaptability
Boost your spirits and get better sleep

Physical Changes to Consider

However, there are a few important things to remember when working out:
As your baby gets bigger, your center of gravity and balance will alter.
Your breathing may become more labored when the needs for oxygen change.
As blood volume rises, so does the workload on your heart.
Hormones related to pregnancy can cause ligaments to stretch and release.

How to Exercise Safely

It's crucial to warm up and cool down before and after an exercise session, whether or not you're expecting. Spend five to ten minutes warming up your muscles and getting your body ready before an activity session. After your workout, take it slow and steady instead of ending all at once. The same type of exercise, such as walking or swimming, can be done during the warm-up and cool-down phases, but it should be done more slowly and at a reduced intensity.

Other crucial advice is as follows:
Wear clothing appropriate for the weather
Put on the proper attire, such as walking shoes with support.
Make sure to stay hydrated.
Consume a balanced, healthful diet.

Safety tips

Avoid going overboard. Avoid working yourself to exhaustion when exercising, and stop if you start to have trouble breathing. You might be jeopardizing the oxygen your developing baby receives if you feel low on oxygen.
Avoid taking chances. Steer clear of anything that can injure your abdomen.
Exercises that require bouncy, jerky actions should be avoided. Steer clear of uterine-compressing workouts.
Avoid lying flat on your back workouts in the second and third trimesters of pregnancy. Reduced oxygen supply and blood flow are linked to this posture.

Warning Indications to Look Out for

If you encounter any of the following, cease exercising and give your doctor a call:
Severe discomfort
Bleeding vaginally
Fluid leakage
Feeling lightheaded or faint
Severe dyspnea

When to Give Up on Exercise

Don't work out if:
You could give birth prematurely.
You have fluid leakage or bleeding.
Your water supply is broken.
Preeclampsia is the term for elevated blood pressure during pregnancy.
You need to be less active due to additional medical conditions or complications.
You're on bedrest.

Chapter Nine

Vegan or Vegetarian and pregnant

It's crucial to eat a healthy diet during pregnancy for both you and the wellbeing of your developing baby.

To ensure that you and your unborn baby receive adequate nutrients for growth and development, it's critical to consume a varied and balanced diet throughout your pregnancy.

Make sure you obtain adequate iron and vitamin B12, which are mostly found in meat and fish, as well as vitamin D, calcium, and iodine, if you're vegetarian or vegan and pregnant.

Iron in your diet

For vegans and vegetarians, dark green vegetables and pulses are good sources of iron.

morning cereals fortified (with additional iron)
with wholemeal bread and flour nuts
dried fruit—apricots, for example

Consuming vitamin B12

Eggs, cheese, and milk are vegetarians'
excellent sources of vitamin B12.
Vegans can benefit from the following sources:
vitamin B12-fortified breakfast cereals;
unsweetened soy beverages; yeast extracts,
such Marmite; and vitamin B12-fortified
nutritional yeast flakes.

Vitamin D in your diet

The majority of people should be able to obtain
adequate vitamin D from sunlight from late
March or early April through the end of
September.

Even though the sunlight provides us with
vitamin D, Vegetarian food sources include:
egg yolk, foods fortified with vitamin D, such as
several breakfast cereals and nutritional
supplements with fat spreads.

It might be challenging to obtain adequate

vitamin D from naturally occurring vitamin D-containing foods and fortified foods on their own because vitamin D is present in few foods.

For this reason, during the winter (October through the end of March), the government advises all adults, including those who are pregnant and nursing, to think about taking a daily supplement containing 10 milligrams of vitamin D.

If you have brown or black skin (for example, if you're of African, African Caribbean, or south Asian descent), cover your skin when you're outside, or spend a lot of time indoors, you may be particularly at risk of not getting enough vitamin D.

You might need to think about taking a vitamin D supplement every day throughout the year.

Consult a physician or midwife for guidance. Make sure your vitamin D is appropriate for vegans if you follow a vegan diet by reading the label.

Calcium in your diet

You also need to make sure you consume adequate calcium if you follow a vegan diet. This is because dairy products provide the majority of calcium for non-vegans.

For vegans, some good sources of calcium are:
Dark green leafy vegetables;
pulses;
unsweetened, fortified soy, pea, and oat beverages
White and brown bread
Tofu with calcium set
Dried fruit with tahini and sesame seeds

See your doctor or midwife about ways to ensure you and your unborn baby are getting all the nutrition you require.

Iodine in your diet

For vegetarians, dairy products, eggs, and cow's milk are good sources of iodine.

Plant foods like cereals and grains also contain

iodine, albeit the amounts differ based on the iodine content of the soil in which the plants are planted.

If you follow a vegan diet, you might want to think about taking an iodine supplement or consuming iodine-fortified foods and some types of plant based drinks.

A one-week sample meal plan

This meal plan includes seven days of high-nutrient vegan foods that will support your pregnancy.

Day 1:

Breakfast: soy milk chia pudding with your choice of nuts, seeds, and fruit on top.

Lunch: quinoa, diced avocados, black beans, roasted peppers, and sunflower seeds served over mixed greens with a drizzle of lemon-basil vinaigrette.

Dinner: whole grain penne pasta served over arugula with a tomato sauce made with tofu or seitan.

Day 2:

Breakfast: Shake of spinach, mango, and oats

Lunch: roasted kale chips, black bean dip, guacamole, and whole grain pita chips with salsa.

Dinner: bok choy, baby corn, peppers, tempeh, rice noodles, and vegan teriyaki sauce stir-fried together.

Day 3:

Breakfast: whole wheat tortilla filled with scrambled tofu, roasted mushrooms, and pesto, along with a soy cappuccino.

Lunch: wakame salad, edamame, vegan miso soup, and vegetable sushi rolls.

Dinner: red lentil dahl over wild rice with spinach, carrots, and broccoli.

Day 4:

Breakfast: overnight oats garnished with fruit, nuts, and seeds.

Lunch: sautéed beet greens on the side and tofu mushroom quiche.

Dinner: roasted sweet potatoes with sautéed collard greens, corn, avocado, tomato sauce, and white beans on top.

Day 5:

Breakfast: Plant yogurt with homemade granola, fresh fruit, nut butter, coconut flakes, and flax seeds .

Lunch: udon noodle soup with tofu and a selection of veggies.

Dinner: cooked amaranth on a bed of black bean and kale chili.

Day 6:

Breakfast: Pancakes with peanut butter, plant yogurt, fruit, and a drizzle of maple syrup

Lunch: Spanish-style tortilla de patatas, which are topped with chopped peppers and greens and cooked with chickpea flour, English potatoes, onions, and black beans.

Dinner: vegetable burger that is completely filled and served with carrot and red cabbage coleslaw.

Day 7:

Breakfast: Homemade vegan blueberry-rosemary scones with nut butter, plant yogurt, fresh fruit, and a glass of fortified orange juice

Lunch: puffed quinoa, shredded red cabbage, white bean pumpkin soup, and coconut milk drizzled on top.

Dinner: radish side salad and vegan lasagna with seitan, eggplant, zucchini, and cashew basil spread.

Healthy pregnancy snacks

Roasted chickpea
Popcorn top with nutritional yeast
Hummus with veggies
Nut butter with fresh fruit
Trail mix
Handmade energizing balls
Homemade muffins
Chia pudding

Edamame
Plant milk with granola

In Summary

All phases of life, including pregnancy, can benefit nutritionally from balanced vegan diets.

Actually, issues including postpartum depression, cesarean delivery, and mother or infant death may be prevented by following a vegan diet.

On the other hand, unplanned vegan diets can raise your baby's development problems, low birth weight, preterm delivery, and vitamin shortages.

As a result, sticking to a vegan diet throughout pregnancy needs meticulous preparation. See a dietician who specializes in plant-based diets to ensure you are meeting your nutritional needs.

Chapter Ten

Labor and Postpartum

Navigating the transition to motherhood A woman's life begins anew as her prenatal journey ends in the life-changing experiences of labor and the postpartum phase. The dynamics of care and well-being change significantly as the body gets ready for the enormous work of birthing and after delivering a new life into the world.

Labor

A Symphony of Strength and Resilience

A woman's body is a living example of strength and resiliency throughout labor. A series of intricate physiological and psychological processes come together to produce the amazing event of giving birth. The journey of labor, from the first contractions to the successful delivery, requires steadfast support, compassion, and most importantly, empowerment.

Aside from the physical elements of contractions and pushing, Labor also requires the mental and emotional strength to face the unknown. Along the way, birthing partners, medical professionals, and the woman herself collaborate to foster an atmosphere of respect, trust, and encouragement. Every labor story is different and reflects the range of experiences that women have worldwide.

Labor Food

Is It Allowed for Me to Eat During Labor?

Of course! Some laboring women experience hunger and thirst, particularly in the early phases of the process. Eating is particularly crucial in the early stages of labor because it will maintain your strength and give you the energy you'll need for the duration of active labor. As you move into more active labor and approach closer to pushing, it's possible that you'll naturally lose the desire to eat. Make sure you consume modest portions of easily digested meals that sound delicious to you at the moment and that you know you like if you are experiencing hunger during active labor.

Select meals that are easy on the stomach and light. Foods high in fat, sugar, or oil are not the best options for labor meals; instead, choose complex carbs.

Food restriction during labor can lead to issues.

Aside from the stress aspects, cutting back on meals during labor can lead to ketosis, which is the state in which the body begins to use its own fat reserves as fuel, and dehydration. It is better to avoid going into ketosis when you have physically demanding tasks ahead of you, as it can cause nausea, vomiting, headaches, and may be an indication of weariness.

Which foods are ideal to eat when going into labor?

When in moderation, it's great to follow your appetite! It's important to keep in mind that eating a lot of fat can make you feel nauseous. Because they provide a prolonged, gradual flow of energy to support you during contractions, carbohydrates are an excellent dietary choice for labor.

Foods to consume during the early stages of labor:

Whole wheat /crackers with seeds
Graham Crackers
Fruit
Wholesome smoothies
Celery, Bananas, and Apples with Almond butter
Whole wheat/ Rice pasta
Miso soup or broth
Yogurt
Tea made from herbs, particularly nettle and raspberry leaf
Pure white grape juice
Popsicles made with real apple juice, ideally handcrafted with natural juices
Juice from natural fruits (not orange juice)
Tea with honey added and frozen into ice cubes
Wholesome cereals
Noodles
Cooked brown rice grains, such as quinoa, millet, and oats
Boiled or scrambled eggs
Applesauce

What should I drink when I'm in labor?

It's crucial to stay hydrated when in labor because labor can be a prolonged, thirst-inducing process. Make an effort to sip on something at least once every hour and every 15 to 30 minutes. Ensure that you always have a drink on hand from one of your labor support assistants. An excellent option is to insert a straw into your drink so that periodically, ideally after every contraction, your partner or doula can hold it to your lips. You will drink if you feel like it and not if you don't. Make sure someone is monitoring your overall fluid consumption. Encouragement to sip water after each contraction is an excellent starting point, and you should strive to drink 1-2 liters of water per hour.

Athletes' go-to isotonic beverages are advised for labor, especially if you're not feeling like eating. Electrolyte powders such as Emergen-C are available at pharmacies. Drinks that are isotonic absorb rapidly and provide your body with the correct kind of energy for strenuous exercise. An excellent option is always filtered water with a squeeze of fresh lemon and a dash of Himalayan rock salt. If not, simply use purified water mixed with diluted apple juice. Orange juice is generally not advised because it may cause nausea or vomiting. Making ice cubes from your preferred fruit juice or smoothie and sucking on them while you labor is a terrific alternative. It's a fantastic substitute for plain water and will provide you with an extra energy boost when you need it. One of the greatest beverages to have during labor is coconut water because it is mild-tasting and rich in electrolytes. Selecting a flavor should be done carefully because you might taste it again and find it unpleasant. Additionally, make sure to stay away from carbonated, sugary drinks.

How would I handle a necessity for a C-section?

The fear that a woman may need a cesarean delivery is what led to the custom of not eating during labor. There is a very small chance that food from the stomach could regurgitate and enter your lungs while you are under general anesthesia. That being said, there is very little chance that this will occur. First off, most cesarean sections performed today do not include general anesthesia. Most are carried out under an epidural or spinal injection, which means you would be awake during the cesarean section. Secondly, the risk is low even in the case of unconsciousness thanks to advances in anesthetic therapy. In order to keep you from breathing in anything from your stomach while you sleep, the anesthetist will apply slight pressure to the cricoid cartilage in your neck, compressing the gullet (esophagus).

Postpartum

 The Start of a New Chapter
Known as the "fourth trimester," the postpartum period is a period of significant changes and learning. A woman welcomes her baby into the world and, at the same time, sets out on a road of healing and adjustment for herself. Postpartum includes the delicate dance of caring for a newborn as well as mental and physical recovery.

The body starts its physical recuperation from the labors and strains of childbirth. Hormones change, muscles heal, and the uterus progressively goes back to how it was before the pregnancy. The postpartum phase can be an emotional rollercoaster of happiness, tiredness, and vulnerability. Support networks, such as friends, family, and medical professionals, are essential to a mother's and her child's wellbeing.

Postpartum life is not just about the struggles and victories in the first few days and weeks after delivery. It entails figuring out how to nurse, creating sleep schedules, and accepting the changing face of parenthood. Self-care becomes a top concern, and getting help from loved ones, support groups, or medical professionals becomes essential to the process.

This delicate tango between childbirth and postpartum is how motherhood is narrated. It's a tale of love, tenacity, and strength that changes with every contraction, the sweet moment of the first hug, and the plethora of events that mold the deep bond between a mother and her child. The pooled knowledge and compassion of communities help women as they set out on this life-changing path, ushering in a stunning and long-lasting chapter in the story of parenthood.

Postpartum Nutrition

A mother's body needs this time to heal from pregnancy and delivery after giving birth.

Prioritize your health by choosing a healthy diet as your body adjusts to the changes brought on by childbirth. Despite the fact that thinking about nutrition in the midst of taking care of a newborn may feel daunting, it's important to make sure your body has the nourishment it needs to heal, adapt, and recover. Here are some thoughts about meals that improve energy, how to balance hormones, the necessity of staying hydrated, and necessary nutrients for postpartum recovery.

Essential Nutrients for Postpartum Recovery

Increased nutritional intake is necessary during the postpartum phase to hasten recovery. A healthy ratio of proteins, lipids, and carbohydrates can aid in the healing process. Choose nutrient-dense foods such as fruits, vegetables, lean meats, nuts, and seeds that are high in fiber, vitamins, minerals, iron, and calcium. Eggs, dairy products, iron-rich seafood, dark leafy greens, and dairy products can help increase energy and decrease weariness.

Hormone Balance with Nutrition

Postpartum hormone imbalances can cause anxiety, despair, and mood swings. Start with a balanced diet to help with hormone balancing. Avoid skipping meals or delaying eating because doing so may result in low blood sugar, which can induce weariness, sadness, and irritability. Include foods high in fiber that are packed with antioxidants, such as berries and whole grains, foods high in Omega-3 fatty acids, such as salmon and sardines, and mood-boosting supplements, such as probiotics, iron, or vitamin D, in your diet.

Staying Hydrated

As your body produces more urine and sweat and as you create breast milk, it is important to stay hydrated. It can also hasten healing and help avoid constipation. Drink water on a regular basis and keep a full bottle close at hand. Drink plenty of nutrient-dense, wholesome liquids to stay hydrated, such as water, coconut water, herbal teas, or freshly squeezed fruit and vegetable juices. Although ten cups of liquids should be

consumed daily as a general rule, keep in mind
that individual needs can differ. Pay attention to
your body's signals; it may need a little more or
a little less. The cues from your body serve as
your compass!

Foods to Fight Postpartum Fatigue

During the postpartum period, especially if you
are sleep deprived, it is common to feel
exhausted. A few high-energy foods to try
include oatmeal, eggs, bananas, nuts and
seeds, brown rice, and leafy greens like kale
and spinach. Due to their high content of vital
vitamins and minerals, these meals can help
increase your energy levels and make it
simpler to do everyday chores.

Nutritional Tips for Nursing Mothers

Approximately 450–500 additional calories per
day are required by nursing mothers in order to
sustain a healthy milk supply and feed their
infants. Three major meals and two to three
nutrient-dense snacks are part of a balanced
breastfeeding diet. Include foods high in
healthy fats, protein, and vitamin B in your diet.
A few ways to accomplish this are to have
yogurt with berries, oatmeal with nuts, milk,

and honey, or a combination of nuts and fruits for breakfast. Including complex carbs, such whole grains, can also provide you with long-lasting energy to start the day.

Getting Help

It's critical to recognize how challenging it might be to focus on postpartum nutrition and adjust to motherhood. Prioritize your own well-being by assigning tasks to others or requesting assistance when required. To focus on your health, ask family or friends for assistance with childcare and domestic duties. You can also speak with a nutritionist, who can help you adjust to this new stage of life by making recommendations that are specific to you.

Although the postpartum period can be difficult, paying attention to your diet can help you feel better overall and make the adjustment easier. Make a deliberate effort to emphasize rest and recuperation, eat meals high in nutrients, and drink enough water. Recall that there are no shortcuts when it comes to healing; it takes time. You may reclaim your health and fully enjoy parenting with perseverance and patience.

Chapter Eleven

Sensitivities and Food allergies

Pregnant women who have food allergies or sensitivities must carefully manage their diets to protect the health and wellbeing of both themselves and their unborn baby. These conditions can provide special obstacles. The following are some things to think about and suggestions for handling food sensitivities and allergies while pregnant:

Food Allergies:

Identify Allergens: It's critical to recognize and stay away from those particular allergens if you have a confirmed food allergy. Peanuts, tree nuts, dairy, eggs, soy, wheat, fish, and shellfish are among the common food allergies.

Examine the labels: Read food labels carefully to be sure there are no potential allergies. Common allergies must be listed prominently on product labels, according to regulations.

Interact with Healthcare Professionals: Tell your medical professionals about any food sensitivities you may have. They can answer questions, offer tailored advice, and make sure that any supplements or prescription drugs don't contain any allergies.

Make Wise Substitutions: Look for acceptable alternatives to allergy-causing items in recipes. If you're allergic to dairy, for instance, look into calcium-rich plant-based milks or leafy greens as substitutes.

Emergency Procedure: Be ready for unintentional exposure. Together with your healthcare professional, go over an emergency plan that includes using an epinephrine auto-injector if needed.

Food Sensitivities

Identify your Triggers: Note any foods that cause sensitivity reactions. This could entail tracking trends and keeping an eye on how you feel after eating particular items.

Typical Sensitivities: Some pregnant women may suffer sensitivities, even if these are not real allergies. Caffeine, spicy and acidic foods, and some foods that cause gas are common triggers. Observe your body's reaction and modify your diet as necessary.

Balanced Diet: Make an effort to eat a diet that is both nutritionally adequate for you and free of things that can aggravate your sensitivity. Seek advice from a dietician if necessary.

Hydration: Drink plenty of water to help with digestion and to ease any discomfort brought on by specific sensitivities.

Small, frequent Meals: To assist control sensitivities like nausea or heartburn, think about eating smaller, more often meals rather than larger ones.

Speak with Medical Professionals:

Registered dietitians with prenatal nutrition expertise should be consulted. They can assist you in creating a diet plan that satisfies your nutritional requirements and is well-balanced.

Assessment by an Allergist: If you suffer from severe allergies, you should think considering seeing an allergist. They can offer you particular advice and take care of any worries you may have about possible allergens in your surroundings.

Frequent Maternal Examinations:
Keep lines of communication open with your healthcare team about any nutritional issues or difficulties you may be experiencing, and schedule regular prenatal checkups.

Every pregnancy is different, so what works for one woman might not work for another. To guarantee that you and your infant get the nutrition you need while successfully managing food allergies and sensitivities during this life-changing time, tailored advice from medical professionals is crucial.

Conclusion

"Real Food for Pregnancy: Nourishing the Journey"
The journey through the complex landscape of maternal nourishment comes to an end in the last pages of "Real Food for Pregnancy," leaving behind a tapestry woven with empowerment, wisdom, and celebration of the fundamental relationship between food and the amazing journey of pregnancy. This book has served as more than just a reference; it has become a friend and a confidante in food, encouraging pregnant mothers to adopt a balanced approach to nutrition.

As the chapters unfolded, the concept of "real food" became apparent as a tenet, supporting the capacity of whole, nutrient-dense ingredients to transform. The story has been one of careful eating, diversity in the kitchen, and an appreciation of the rich flavors and textures that sustain both body and soul—from the foundational stages of the first trimester to the thrilling moments of labor and the delicate dance of postpartum recovery.

Beyond just offering standard nutritional advice, the book encourages readers to consider pregnancy as a whole and delicious experience rather than just a physical journey. It has examined the subtleties of customizing diets to the distinct phases of pregnancy, encouraging pregnant mothers to customize their intake in accordance with their own tastes, cultural influences, and evolving requirements.

The book has shed light on the critical roles that many nutrients, such as folic acid, iron, calcium, and omega-3 fatty acids, play in the complex dance between fetal development and maternal health. It has helped to deconstruct the science surrounding these nutrients and promote a shift away from supplements and toward the full range of tastes that come from real, wholesome foods.

"Real Food for Pregnancy" is, at its core, a celebration of the wonders of new life, the tenacious resilience of women, and the transforming potential of thoughtful, delicious food. In addition to imparting a plethora of nutritional knowledge, it also gives its readers a sense of empowerment by showing them how to face parenthood with courage, fortitude, and a profound understanding of the relationship between real food and the remarkable chapters of pregnancy.

As the book comes to a conclusion, it leaves behind a legacy: an invitation to appreciate the wisdom of the body, to taste the richness of real food, and to approach pregnancy with a spirit of nourishment that goes well beyond the plate. The journey of embracing, relishing, and appreciating the flavors of pregnancy lingers even after the pages close, reiterating the age-old adage that real food is more than simply nourishment; it's a celebration of life.